THE QUIET BATTLEFIELD

MATT MCVEY ARROWOOD

THE QUIET BATTLEFIELD

MATT MCVEY ARROWOOD

This book is dedicated to all service members past, present, and future. Thank you for your service and thank you for reading!!!!

CHAPTER 1

HOMECOMING

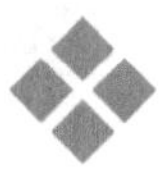

Tom Cross stepped off the plane and into the waiting area as he breathed in the sterile air of the airport. It had been almost two years since he'd last set foot on American soil, but somehow it felt longer, as if he left decades ago and came back a different man but then maybe he had. The weight of his duffle bag strained his shoulder, pressing into scar tissue he'd grown used to, and he adjusted it automatically, his mind half-frozen with exhaustion and anticipation.

He scanned the small crowd waiting near the terminal, seeing faces blurred together in one anxious, unfamiliar sea. His mother was easy to spot, her short gray hair like a beacon in the crowd. Next to her, his dad stood stiffly, hands in his pockets, looking more nervous than Tom had ever seen him. A few steps back, his sister Rachel waved, her face a mix of forced excitement and… was it worry? It had been so long since he'd seen them that he couldn't be sure anymore.

As he approached, his mother's face softened into a smile that didn't reach her eyes, and she wrapped him in a hug. He forced himself to hug back, though his mind was somewhere else, back on the tarmac, back in the hot, choking air of another country, another world.

"We're so happy you're home, Tommy," she whispered, her voice catching.

"Good to be back," he lied. The words felt hollow, hanging in the air between them.

His father shook his hand firmly, a formality that reminded Tom of high school graduation or the day he'd first left for basic training. His dad's face was lined and weary, eyes slightly narrowed as he looked Tom over, searching for… something. Tom wasn't sure what. A version of himself that had died over there, maybe.

"Let's get you home," his dad said finally, clapping a hand on Tom's shoulder. The weight of it felt strange, almost foreign. Tom nodded, keeping his face blank, focusing on the simple movement of walking, one step after the other.

The drive home was quiet, punctuated by his mother's soft questions. "How was the flight?" "Are you hungry?" "Do you need to rest?" He answered each one mechanically, realizing with a pang that he barely knew how to talk to them anymore. They hadn't been a part of his life out there, not in the way the men beside him had been. His family had been letters, fleeting phone calls, and muffled voices from another world, disconnected from the dust, the heat, and the sounds that had become his everyday life.

When they reached the house, Tom took in the familiar sight: the brick-fronted two-story home he'd grown up in, the modest yard, the weathered porch swing that creaked when the wind blew. He'd always thought he'd be happy to see it again. Now, it felt distant, like something from someone else's memory.

Inside, the living room was unchanged, with the same photographs on the wall, the same worn couches and hand-me-down furniture. Right down to the cigarette burns, from where his mother used to smoke. His mother had set up a small welcome-home banner across the entryway, a pitiful, brightly-colored thing that clashed with the dark suitcases at his feet.

He glanced around, noting the missing faces. His uncle and cousins hadn't come, probably out of respect for his "adjustment period," or so his dad had said over the phone. But Tom suspected they just didn't know how to greet him, the man who had come back instead of the boy who'd left. It didn't matter. He wasn't in a rush to reconnect. The family had done what they could with the limited information they had, throwing him a welcome-home party that felt like a stranger's attempt at comfort.

Rachel nudged him gently. "Tom, are you good?" she asked, her voice barely a whisper.

He nodded, forcing a tight smile. "Yeah, Rach. Just tired."

She smiled back, though her eyes searched his face with the same careful, guarded curiosity his parents wore. Everyone seemed to be looking for something, some reassurance that he was okay, that he was Tom, the brother and son who had left. But that Tom was gone, or buried so deep he wasn't sure he'd ever find him again.

As the evening wore on, they danced around questions they clearly wanted to ask, questions he had no answers for. They talked about the neighbors, about Rachel's new job, about our cousin's wedding. He went through the motions, nodding and smiling, but his mind was elsewhere, drifting back to the humid nights and sand-swept days of his last deployment.

The unease set in deep, a steady pressure in his chest. He felt like a ghost walking through his own life, passing through rooms that held memories he couldn't reach. Every attempt at normal conversation only heightened the growing distance between him and his family, a rift he wasn't sure how to bridge.

When he finally made it to his old room, he shut the door and sank onto the bed, the faint smell of stale linens filling his senses. He closed his eyes, breathing deeply, his mind racing with images he didn't want to see. Faces, moments, the sounds of home giving way to sounds he'd tried to leave behind.

His fingers twitched, instinctively reaching for a bottle that wasn't there. He cursed under his breath, feeling the sudden and all-consuming pull of alcohol as the only thing that could blur the edges of the memories. The craving clawed at him, a reminder that while he may have left the battlefield, the fight was far from over.

CHAPTER 2

GHOSTS OF THE PAST

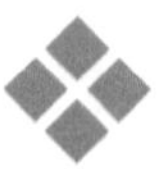

The days following Tom's return home slipped by, each one blurring into the next. Every morning, he woke up in his old bedroom, and for a brief, disorienting moment, he expected to hear the distant sounds of choppers or the sharp crackle of a radio. But all he heard was the dull hum of the air conditioning and the creak of the house settling. His parents tried to keep him busy, filling the quiet with family dinners and neighborhood updates. His sister Rachel stopped by whenever she could, bringing stories of her work and her friends. They all seemed to think if they just kept talking, it would somehow pull him back into civilization.

He went through the motions, responding with polite nods and forced smiles. But every conversation only reminded him of how far he'd drifted from them, from himself. It felt like his family was tiptoeing around him, measuring their words and watching his reactions. They seemed afraid to ask him anything real, afraid of what he might say, or maybe of what he wouldn't say.

One night, unable to sleep, Tom sat on the edge of his bed, scrolling through his phone contacts. He stopped at a name that felt like it belonged to another life: David Haynes. They'd enlisted together and gone through basic side by side. Out of everyone Tom served with, David had been the one he'd stayed closest to. David was still in touch with the old unit, still connected to that world Tom had left behind.

Without thinking too much, Tom tapped the number and held the phone to his ear. It rang a few times before a familiar voice picked up.

"Tom?" David's voice was both surprised and cautious. "Man, it's been a while."

"Yeah, it has," Tom replied, surprised by how rough his own voice sounded. "Just…thought I'd check in."

David chuckled, but there was an edge to it. "Well, glad you called. I was starting to think you'd gone off the grid or something."

They exchanged a few pleasantries, trading stories about old friends, and for a moment, Tom felt a faint sense of comfort, like he was slipping back into an old rhythm. But the comfort was short-lived. As they talked, he realized how much he had changed. David sounded the same, his laugh easy, his voice steady. David still had his job, his family. He talked about his wife's latest project, the new car he'd just bought. Tom could barely relate.

"So, how's the leg?" David asked, after a pause.

Tom tensed, a reflex he couldn't quite shake. He looked down at his knee, the joint stiff and aching, wrapped in a brace that he'd grown to resent. "It's…fine. Doctors say I'll be walking normally soon. Might even get back into running." It was a half-truth at best, but he couldn't bring himself to admit that even walking without pain was still a ways off.

David paused, as though weighing his words. "You know, Tom…if you ever need to talk about it, I mean, about what happened…"

Tom cut him off before he could finish. "I'm fine, Dave," he said, forcing a bit too much conviction into his voice. "Just trying to settle back in, you know? Get back to normal."

But what did normal even mean anymore?

David cleared his throat, and Tom could feel the awkwardness thickening between them. "Yeah, man. I get it. Just…take care of yourself, alright? Don't be a stranger."

After they hung up, Tom sat in the quiet, his phone still clutched in his hand. Talking to David should have been a relief, but instead, it left him feeling more isolated than ever. David had been his closest friend out there, the one person who understood what they'd gone through. But now, even he felt like a stranger.

The following days were even harder. His family tried to pull him back into routines, and Tom tried to keep up the facade of normalcy. But every familiar sight, every trivial conversation, felt like an echo of something he'd left behind.

He tried to fill his days with small tasks, chores around the house, anything to keep busy. But his thoughts drifted constantly, pulled back to memories he couldn't shake.

One afternoon, while clearing out his old room, he came across a box he hadn't seen in years. Inside were pieces of his life before the army: high school yearbooks, a few dusty soccer trophies, and a stack of old photographs. He thumbed through them, pausing at a picture of himself and David, grinning and flushed, in their first month of basic. They looked so young, so certain of what they were doing. He could almost feel the weight of his old uniform, the thrill of those first few weeks, before reality had settled in.

He dropped the photo back in the box, feeling a surge of frustration rise in his chest. All these pieces of his old life didn't mean anything now. He slammed the lid shut and shoved the box back under his bed, feeling the familiar tug of frustration and anger beneath his ribs.

That night, he lay in bed, wide awake, his mind replaying scenes he wished he could forget. Faces, names, sounds that crept into his mind and refused to leave. He could almost hear the low hum of the desert air, the distant echo of gunfire. The walls around him seemed to close in, pressing him back to places he'd left, places he could never truly escape.

By midnight, the craving for something to numb the noise became unbearable. He went to the kitchen, opening and closing the fridge, staring blankly at the rows of soda cans and bottles of juice that his mom had stocked. He could almost feel the bite of whiskey against his throat, the way it dulled the edges of his thoughts, turning memories into something softer, something easier to ignore.

But there was nothing there. His parents had cleared the house of alcohol the day he'd arrived, a silent gesture of support or maybe it was a warning, he wasn't sure. He clenched his fists, shutting the fridge and leaning against the counter, breathing heavily, trying to calm the storm inside.

He knew he couldn't keep going like this, trapped between the world he'd left and the one he didn't recognize anymore. He'd tried to reach out to David, tried to reconnect, but it had only driven home the truth: there was no one who could pull him out of this. Not David, not his family. He was on his own, facing battles they couldn't see, battles he barely understood himself.

As he stood there in the quiet kitchen, he realized he was back in a different kind of war zone, one that couldn't be left behind with a plane ride home. And this time, he wasn't sure he had the strength to fight it.

CHAPTER 3

THE SPIRAL

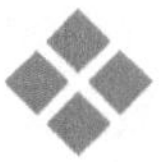

Tom's days slipped into a pattern of restless nights and numbing routines. He'd wake up late, sometimes to the sound of his mother calling him for breakfast, though most days he'd tell her he'd "eat later." He'd drink coffee alone in the kitchen, staring out the window at the quiet street he used to know so well, wondering how everything could feel so far away. The whole world seemed muted, like he was on the other side of a thick pane of glass.

Without a job or a plan, he filled his days with pointless tasks. He'd go for long drives without a destination, circling the town aimlessly until he found himself at old spots he used to visit. Sometimes he'd sit outside the bar downtown, watching people come and go. Watching them drink, laugh, talk with ease. He'd sit there, just out of sight, feeling like an outsider to a life he'd never fit back into.

The drinking started slowly. At first, he convinced himself it was just one or two beers to take the edge off. But those beers turned into whiskey, and the whiskey turned into nights he couldn't remember. Nights he barely wanted to. It was like turning down the volume on everything, letting the noise and the memories fade into a dull buzz. In those hazy moments, it almost felt like peace.

But peace never lasted. The morning would come, and he'd wake up with a pounding headache and a gnawing emptiness that felt even worse than before. His mother noticed, of course her glances became sharper, her voice more strained when she spoke to him. She'd never ask him outright, but she didn't need to. Her silence said it all. She was watching him unravel, and he didn't know how to stop it.

One night, after a few too many shots at a bar downtown, Tom found himself stumbling through the parking lot, his mind hazy and numb. He could barely remember how he'd gotten there, only that he needed another drink, something to keep the memories away. But as he fumbled for his keys, he heard a voice call his name.

"Tom? Tom Cross?"

He turned, squinting in the dim light, and recognized a familiar face. Steve, an old high school classmate, one of the guys he'd played soccer with. Steve looked at him with a mixture of surprise and pity, like he'd just found a ghost.

"Didn't know you were back in town," Steve said, his voice careful.

"Yeah," Tom mumbled, trying to keep his balance. "Back a few weeks now."

Steve's eyes flicked down to the bottle in Tom's hand, and his expression hardened. "Hey, maybe you should let me call you a cab. You don't look too steady."

Tom's face twisted in frustration. "I'm fine," he snapped, though his voice was slurred. "Don't need no babysitter."

But Steve didn't back down. "Look, man, it's not a big deal. Let me just call someone, alright? You don't want to drive like this."

At that moment, something snapped in Tom. He'd spent weeks feeling like an outsider, barely able to connect with anyone. And here was Steve, trying to play the hero, trying to tell him what to do, as if he understood a fraction of what Tom had been through. The frustration boiled over, and before he knew it, his fists were clenched, his voice rising.

"Don't tell me what I can and can't do, alright?" he shouted, the anger pouring out of him. "You don't know anything about me, about what I've been through. So don't stand there and act like you're doing me a favor."

Steve raised his hands, stepping back. "Alright, Tom. Take it easy. I'm just trying to help."

But Tom didn't want help. Not from Steve, not from anyone. The rage inside him felt bigger than he was, like it would swallow him whole if he didn't get away. So he stumbled to his truck, ignoring Steve's protests, and drove off into the night, his vision blurring as the lights of the town flashed past him.

The next morning, he woke up to the blinding pain of a hangover and the sharp taste of regret. His mother was waiting in the kitchen, her arms crossed and her face drawn tight.

"We need to talk," she said, her voice low and steady.

He braced himself, knowing what was coming.

She gestured to the kitchen table, where a glass of water and a small, crumpled note lay. "Steve called," she said, her voice trembling slightly. "He was worried about you, and said you were in bad shape last night."

Tom looked away, the shame pressing down on him. "It was nothing. Just a rough night."

His mother's face softened, her eyes filling with concern. "Tom, you can't keep doing this to yourself. You came back to us… but it feels like we're losing you all over again."

He swallowed, the words stinging. "I'm fine, Mom. I can handle it."

But she didn't back down. "Can you? Because it doesn't seem like it. You won't talk to us, you won't let us in. And every night, you disappear and come back…like this!" Her voice broke, and she looked away, her hands clenched tightly on the edge of the table. As Tom looked at her he realized that she had started to cry.

For a moment, he wanted to reach out, to tell her everything, to let her see the weight he carried. But he couldn't. The words caught in his throat, tangled with pride and fear and anger. He couldn't tell her what he'd seen, what he couldn't unsee. He couldn't explain the nightmares that crept in whenever he closed his eyes. It was just too much and he didn't want anyone else to have to bear any of the weight, especially his mother.

Instead, he mumbled an apology, hating himself for the hollow sound of it. She nodded, though he could see the hurt in her eyes. She left him alone in the kitchen, the silence settling around him like a shroud.

As he sat there, he felt the walls closing in, the memories crowding his mind. Faces, names, moments he'd tried to bury. He knew he was falling apart, but he didn't know how to stop it. Every night, he drank to forget, but the forgetting only lasted so long. Each morning, the memories came back sharper, cutting deeper.

He felt trapped, caught between the life he'd left and the one he couldn't quite reenter. And every night, the alcohol felt like the only thing that could quiet the noise, even if just for a little while.

As he sat there, he felt the weight of his choices pressing down on him, the ache in his chest a constant reminder of the emptiness he couldn't fill. He didn't know how to face his family, didn't know how to find his way back to them. All he

knew was that he couldn't go on like this. But he didn't know
how to stop, either.

And somewhere, deep down, he wondered if he ever
would.

CHAPTER 4

BREAKING POINT

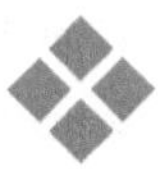

The days grew colder, and the last hints of autumn drifted away as winter crept in. Tom hardly noticed the change. He was numb to almost everything now, moving through his days with a heaviness that weighed down his every step. He avoided family dinners, leaving the house whenever he could, wandering aimlessly, finding himself back in the bars more nights than not.

His family had started to pull back. Rachel didn't stop by as often, and his mother had long since given up on trying to coax him into conversations. His father had barely said a word to him since that morning in the kitchen, their silence settling like a quiet truce built on avoidance. Tom knew they wanted to help him. But he also knew they were tired, worn down by his silence and self-destruction, unsure how to reach him.

One night, after a particularly rough stretch of drinking, he stumbled into the house well past midnight, the air thick with the smell of whiskey. He nearly tripped over his mother's armchair, the light from the hallway catching his eye. To his surprise, his father was sitting there, his face set in a hard line.

"Tom," his father said, his voice low but unwavering. "We need to talk."

Tom sighed, slumping against the doorframe. "I'm tired, Dad. Can we just…not do this right now?"

His father's gaze didn't falter. "You think we're not tired too? You think we haven't been worried every night, wondering if you'll come home in one piece?"

Tom looked away, the shame rising in his throat, but he bit back his anger. "I'm handling it. Just let me…let me deal with it in my own way."

His father stood up, crossing the room in slow, measured steps. "Drinking yourself into oblivion isn't handling it, Tom. It's barely surviving. We've done everything we can to support you, but you're pushing us all away."

Tom clenched his fists, feeling the frustration and helplessness swirl inside him. "You wouldn't understand," he muttered, hating the way his voice sounded weak, defeated.

"Then help us understand," his father said, his voice softening for the first time. "You're not alone, Tom. But if you keep going like this, you will be. You're going to push everyone away, including yourself."

The words hit him like a punch. His father's gaze didn't waver, and Tom could see the pain etched into his face, the desperation of a man who didn't know how to save his own son. In that moment, Tom felt his own defenses crumble, the weight of everything he'd been carrying threatening to pull him under.

But instead of letting himself feel it, he turned and stormed out of the room, his fists clenched as he tried to push down the ache in his chest. He left the house, the cold night air hitting him like a slap, but he barely felt it. He drove until he found himself back at the bar, drowning his thoughts in drink after drink, desperate to numb the shame and guilt.

The next morning, he woke up in his truck, parked haphazardly outside the bar, his head pounding and his mouth dry. The memories of the night before were blurry, but the argument with his father replayed in his mind like a broken record. He wanted to push it away, to ignore the sting of truth in his father's words, but they lingered, gnawing at him.

He drove home, feeling the weight of exhaustion settle over him like a heavy blanket. When he walked inside, he found his mother sitting at the kitchen table, a letter clutched in her hands. She looked up at him, her face lined with worry and sadness.

"Tom, we can't keep doing this," she said, her voice barely above a whisper. "I found a brochure for a veterans' support group. They meet every week at the community center. Please…just consider it."

Tom clenched his jaw, the defensiveness flaring up instantly. "A support group? You really think sitting around with a bunch of strangers is going to fix anything?"

Her eyes softened, and she reached out, placing a hand on his arm. "I don't know, Tom. But I know that what you're doing isn't working. I know that you're hurting, and that you're pushing everyone who loves you away. We just want to see you try, even if it's just this once."

He pulled away, the anger boiling up, though he wasn't even sure who he was angry at. His parents, for not understanding? The military, for sending him home broken? Or himself, for not being able to cope? But beneath the anger was something else, a fear he couldn't ignore, a nagging voice that told him his mother was right.

He nodded stiffly, feeling the words slip out before he could stop them. "Fine. I'll go. Just once."

Her face softened with relief, and she gave his arm a squeeze. "Thank you."

That evening, Tom found himself in the community center, sitting in a circle of folding chairs. The room was filled with men and women of all ages, each wearing the same weary expressions, the same guarded looks that he recognized in himself. He felt out of place, exposed, as if every one of them could see the cracks he'd tried so hard to hide.

The leader of the group, a retired Marine named Carl, started the session by sharing his own story how he'd struggled to adapt to civilian life, how he'd lost friends, and how he'd found himself turning to alcohol to numb the pain. As he spoke, Tom felt a flicker of recognition, a glimmer of understanding. For the first time, he realized he wasn't as alone as he'd thought.

When it was his turn to speak, he felt his throat tighten, the words sticking in his chest. He wanted to keep it short, to say something polite and non-committal, but as he looked around the room, he saw the same pain reflected in their faces. And for the first time, he felt a flicker of something else, something close to hope.

"I...don't really know why I'm here," he said, his voice barely above a whisper. "I guess I thought I could handle things on my own. But...I can't. And I don't know how to fix it."

The words felt raw, like tearing open an old wound, but he forced himself to keep talking, to let them see the parts of him he'd kept hidden. As he spoke, he felt the weight of his pain and anger begin to ease, if only slightly. He didn't know if this was the solution, if this group could truly help him. But for the first time, he felt a small sliver of relief, a crack in the walls he'd built around himself.

When he finished, Carl nodded, his expression one of understanding. "We all thought we could handle it on our own, Tom. But none of us were meant to carry this weight alone."

The rest of the session passed in a blur, each person sharing their story, their own battles. As he listened, Tom felt a connection he hadn't felt in months, a reminder that he wasn't the only one fighting to find his way back. And by the end of the meeting, he found himself promising to return, a promise he didn't know if he'd keep, but one he was willing to try.

That night, for the first time in months, he slept soundly, his dreams quieter, the memories softened around the edges. And as he drifted off, he felt a glimmer of something he hadn't felt in a long time, a sense of hope, fragile and tentative, but real.

CHAPTER 5

THE FIRST STEP

The following week, Tom found himself back at the community center, though he wasn't entirely sure why. He'd spent the past few days thinking of every reason not to return telling himself the group couldn't change anything, that he could handle things his own way. But there was a part of him, a small, tentative part, that clung to the memory of that night, of the strange sense of relief he'd felt after speaking. So he went, hoping that maybe, just maybe, it might help again.

The meeting room was quiet when he arrived, a few familiar faces nodding in recognition as he took his seat. Carl, the leader, gave him a nod and a slight smile, a silent gesture of welcome. Tom settled into his chair, feeling a little less out of place this time. The faces around him were still strangers, but he no longer felt the need to put up the same walls. He'd seen their pain, and they'd seen his. That was enough.

As the session began, Carl introduced a new member, a young woman named Julia who had recently returned from her own deployment. She spoke with a kind of nervous energy, her hands twisting in her lap as she shared her story. Tom watched her, recognizing the same haunted look he saw in the mirror each morning, the same struggle to reconcile the person she'd become with the person she'd once been.

When it was Tom's turn to speak, he hesitated, the familiar impulse to stay silent bubbling up. But then he remembered his mother's face, the sadness in her eyes, the way she'd asked him to try. And so he began to talk, letting the words come out in pieces, sharing a bit more than he had before. He talked about the guilt, the endless nights spent reliving moments he wished he could forget. He didn't say everything not yet but he said enough to feel the weight lift just a little.

By the end of the meeting, he felt a small sense of accomplishment, a feeling he hadn't had in a long time. As the group began to disperse, Carl approached him, clapping a hand on his shoulder.

"You did good today, Tom," he said, his voice steady and reassuring. "Keep showing up. That's half the battle."

Tom nodded, the words sinking in. He didn't know if he'd ever fully open up, if he'd ever share the darkest parts of himself with these people. But he could keep showing up. That much he could do.

The days passed slowly, each one feeling a little more manageable than the last. Tom's family noticed the change, though none of them said anything outright. His mother's worried glances softened, and his father's silence became less tense, less heavy with unspoken words. Even Rachel stopped by more often, her laughter filling the house in a way that reminded Tom of better days.

But the progress was fragile. Each morning, he fought the urge to reach for the bottle, the temptation to slip back into the numbness that had become so familiar. Some days, he won the battle. Other days, he didn't. But each time he slipped, he reminded himself of the group, of Carl's words. Keep showing up. That was all he could do.

One evening, as he sat alone in his room, he found himself staring at an old photo on his dresser. It was from his first deployment—a group shot of him and his squad, all of them smiling, arms slung over each other's shoulders, young and full of purpose. They'd been a family in their own way, bound by experiences no one else could understand. Looking at their faces, Tom felt the familiar ache of loss, the weight of memories he couldn't shake.

He reached for his phone, his fingers hovering over the screen. He hadn't kept in touch with many of them—most had drifted away, finding their own ways to cope with the weight of their experiences. But there was one number he still had, a friend named Jackson who had been there through the worst of it, who had seen Tom at his lowest.

After a moment's hesitation, he dialed the number, his heart pounding as the phone rang. He half-expected Jackson not to pick up, to let it go to voicemail. But then there was a click, and Jackson's voice came through, surprised but familiar.

"Tom? Man, is that you?"

Tom swallowed, the words catching in his throat. "Yeah… it's me."

There was a pause, and then Jackson's tone softened. "Been a long time, buddy. How've you been?"

The question hung heavy in the air, and for a moment, Tom didn't know how to answer. How could he sum up everything he'd been through, the darkness and the struggle, in a few words? But then he remembered the group, the feeling of connection he'd found there, and he decided to be honest.

"I'm…not great," he admitted, the words feeling both painful and liberating. "It's been rough. Really rough."

Jackson was silent for a moment, but when he spoke, his voice was filled with understanding. "I hear you, man. It's not easy. I've been there too."

They talked for a while, sharing stories, memories of their time together, moments of both laughter and pain. For the first time in a long time, Tom felt a sense of connection to his past, a reminder of the person he'd been before everything had gone wrong. By the time they hung up, he felt a small glimmer of something he hadn't felt in a long time… hope.

In the following weeks, Tom continued attending the group, each session feeling a little less daunting than the last. He spoke more openly, sharing bits and pieces of his story, letting himself be vulnerable in a way he'd never allowed before. The group became a lifeline, a place where he could lay down his burdens, even if only for an hour each week.

His relationship with his family began to heal as well, the tension easing with each passing day. His mother's smiles came more easily, his father's voice less strained. Rachel even convinced him to join her for a hike one weekend, something he hadn't done since he'd returned. They walked in silence for much of the trail, but it was a comfortable silence, one filled with an understanding that didn't need words.

One night, after a particularly long group session, Tom found himself sitting in his truck, staring up at the night sky. He thought about everything he'd been through, the battles he'd fought both overseas and within himself. He knew he still had a long way to go, that the road ahead would be filled with setbacks and challenges. But for the first time, he felt a sense of acceptance, a willingness to confront his pain rather than run from it.

As he sat there, he realized something else, he wasn't alone. He had his family, his friends, and the support of others who understood his struggle. And though he still had his doubts, still felt the weight of his past pressing down on him, he knew he had people who would help him carry it.

And for the first time in a long time, that was enough.

CHAPTER 6

SUPPORT AND STRAIN

Tom had been going to the group meetings for a month now. Each time he showed up, he felt a little less out of place, a little less like he was an outsider. He'd gotten to know a few people there: Julia, the young woman who'd just returned from deployment; Carl, the group leader, who always seemed to know when to speak and when to listen; and a man named Ray, an older veteran who'd been through more battles than Tom could imagine.

The group had become a kind of lifeline. There, he could speak openly about the pain, the memories, the constant fight to stay sober. He didn't have to hide anything or pretend to be fine. And for the first time, he felt like he was making progress, like he was clawing his way out of the dark pit he'd been trapped in since he'd come home.

But as he found support in the group, he began to notice the strain his struggles had put on the people closest to him, especially his family.

One evening, he returned home after a particularly intense session, his mind heavy with the stories he'd heard, the emotions he'd shared. Rachel was sitting on the porch steps, wrapped in a sweater, her face turned up to the evening sky. She looked peaceful, almost lost in her own world, and for a moment, Tom hesitated, unsure if he should interrupt her.

But then she looked over and smiled, patting the spot next to her. "Come sit with me, big brother."

He joined her, feeling the cool night air settle around them. They sat in silence for a while, watching the stars come out one by one, neither of them speaking. Tom had always felt a closeness with Rachel, even before the army. They'd been each other's confidants growing up, sharing secrets and inside jokes. But since he'd come home, that closeness had faded, replaced by an unspoken tension he couldn't quite bridge.

After a few minutes, Rachel broke the silence. "You seem…different lately," she said, her voice soft but steady. "In a good way, I mean."

Tom nodded, unsure how to respond. "I'm trying, Rach. It's…hard. But I'm trying."

She glanced at him, her face filled with a mix of relief and lingering worry. "I know. And I'm proud of you for that. We all are. But, Tom…" She hesitated, her fingers twisting together in her lap. "You don't know how hard it was for us, watching you go through all this. There were days when I didn't even recognize you."

Her words hit him like a punch, and he felt a wave of shame wash over him. He'd been so focused on his own pain, his own struggle, that he hadn't considered how it had affected the people who loved him.

"I'm sorry," he murmured, his voice barely above a whisper. "I didn't mean to…hurt you. Any of you."

Rachel reached out, placing a hand on his shoulder. "I know, Tom. And I get that you've been through things I can't even imagine. But you don't have to face it all alone. We're here for you. We always have been."

He nodded, swallowing past the lump in his throat. He'd always thought of himself as strong, as someone who didn't need help. But sitting there with his sister, he realized that maybe strength wasn't about facing everything alone. Maybe it was about allowing himself to lean on the people who cared about him.

They sat together in comfortable silence for a while, the weight of unspoken words settling between them, and Tom felt a sense of peace he hadn't felt in a long time.

In the following days, Tom continued attending his group meetings, each session peeling back another layer of the pain he'd buried deep inside. He grew closer to Julia, who shared her own struggles with adapting to civilian life. She was a few years younger than him, but they shared a bond, an understanding born from their shared experiences.

One afternoon, after a particularly rough session, they decided to grab coffee together. Sitting across from her in the quiet coffee shop, Tom felt a sense of ease that surprised him. For once, he didn't feel the need to put on a mask, to pretend he was fine. Julia understood without him having to explain, and that understanding was a kind of balm he hadn't realized he needed.

They talked about everything: their families, their memories, the constant struggle to find their place in a world that felt alien. Julia was honest about her own battles, admitting to nights spent alone, fighting the same cravings, the same memories. Her openness made Tom feel less alone, and for the first time, he felt like he was making a real connection, one that wasn't built on pity or obligation.

At one point, Julia looked at him, her eyes filled with a quiet intensity. "You know, Tom, we're all damaged in some way. But that doesn't mean we're broken. Sometimes, it just means we need to find new ways to put ourselves back together."

Her words stuck with him, echoing in his mind long after they'd finished their coffee and gone their separate ways. He thought about his family, the people in his support group, and the ways they were all trying to put themselves back together, piece by piece. Maybe that was all anyone could do, keep trying, keep showing up, even when it felt impossible.

As Tom's relationships with his family and support group deepened, he began to feel the weight of his recovery in a new way. He'd always thought of himself as the only one who'd been affected by his experiences, the only one carrying the weight. But now, he saw the truth: his pain had radiated outward, touching the lives of everyone around him.

It was a humbling realization, one that left him feeling both guilty and grateful. He hadn't chosen this path, and hadn't wanted the burden of recovery. But he knew now that he owed it to himself and to those who loved him to keep going.

He still had bad days, days when the memories felt too heavy, when the urge to numb the pain became almost unbearable. But each time, he reminded himself of the people who were standing by him, the people who'd refused to give up on him even when he'd given up on himself.

One evening, after a particularly difficult day, he found himself back on the porch, staring up at the night sky. He thought about Julia's words, about the idea of being damaged but not broken. It was a small distinction, but it felt monumental.

As he sat there, he felt a sense of determination settle over him, a quiet resolve to keep going, to keep fighting. He didn't know what the future held, didn't know if he'd ever truly find peace. But for the first time, he felt like he was on the right path.

He wasn't healed, not by a long shot. But he was healing. And that, he realized, was enough.

CHAPTER 7

FINDING PURPOSE

It was a quiet Thursday afternoon when Carl approached Tom after their usual support group meeting. Tom was packing up, gathering his coat and notebook, his mind still lingering on the stories they'd shared that day. The group had discussed the difficulties of reintegration, the feeling of not belonging anywhere, of drifting without a sense of direction.

Carl placed a hand on Tom's shoulder, a warm, steadying gesture. "Got a minute, Tom?"

"Of course," Tom replied, surprised but curious. Carl's expression was thoughtful, a hint of something serious in his eyes.

"I've noticed you've been making real progress here," Carl said. "I know it hasn't been easy, but you're showing up, sharing, and helping others just by being here. That's something not everyone can do."

Tom shrugged, feeling a mix of pride and self-doubt. "I'm just trying to stay above water, Carl."

"I get that," Carl said, smiling. "But sometimes, the best way to keep your head above water is to help pull someone else up. We're organizing an outreach event next week for veterans in the area. We'll be offering resources, information on support services, and a place for people to connect. I thought maybe you'd want to help out."

Tom felt a flicker of surprise, followed by a familiar pang of doubt. He'd always thought of himself as the one needing help, the one barely holding it together. But Carl's suggestion planted a new idea in his mind, one that felt both daunting and oddly exhilarating.

"You really think I could help?" he asked, his voice barely above a whisper.

Carl's gaze was steady, filled with a quiet certainty. "I know you can. Sometimes, the best people to guide others are the ones who've been through the same darkness. Think about it, alright?"

Tom nodded, the idea taking root, growing into something that felt both terrifying and right. He'd spent so long focusing on his own pain, his own struggles, that he hadn't considered the possibility that he could help others. The thought stayed with him, lingering in his mind as he drove home, replaying Carl's words over and over.

The following week, Tom found himself at the community center, setting up tables and arranging stacks of pamphlets and information sheets. He wasn't sure what to expect, but he felt a strange sense of purpose, a quiet determination to be there for others in a way he hadn't allowed himself before.

The event began, and veterans from around the area trickled in, each one carrying their own invisible weight. Tom recognized some of the faces, people who had come to the support group once or twice before disappearing again. Others were new, cautious and guarded, their eyes wary as they scanned the room.

Throughout the afternoon, Tom spoke with several people, sharing bits of his story and listening to theirs. He was surprised by how natural it felt, how easily the words came. He didn't need to offer solutions or answers; sometimes, just listening was enough. In their shared silences, he found a sense of connection, a reminder that he wasn't alone in his struggles.

At one point, he noticed a young man standing near the door, his hands shoved deep into his pockets, his gaze fixed on the floor. He looked barely out of his teens, his face drawn and weary, like he'd been carrying a heavy burden for far too long. Tom approached him, sensing the familiar tension, the quiet desperation hidden beneath his guarded expression.

"Hey," Tom said, keeping his voice calm and steady. "I'm Tom. Mind if I join you?"

The young man glanced up, nodding slightly. "Sure. Name's Ben."

They stood in silence for a moment, and Tom waited, giving Ben the space to speak if he wanted to. After a few minutes, Ben sighed, his shoulders slumping as he let out a breath he'd been holding.

"I, uh… I didn't know if I'd come," Ben admitted, his voice barely audible. "I've never been to one of these things before. Feels…weird."

Tom nodded, understanding the hesitation all too well. "Yeah, I get that. I didn't think this kind of thing was for me either. But…sometimes, talking to people who understand helps. Even if it's just for a little while."

Ben glanced at him, a flicker of curiosity in his eyes. "Did it help you?"

Tom thought about it, about the months he'd spent trying to claw his way out of the darkness, about the group, the connections he'd made, the small victories he'd managed to hold on to. "Yeah," he said finally. "It didn't fix everything, but it helped. And sometimes, that's enough."

They continued talking, Ben gradually opening up, sharing pieces of his own story, his struggle to find a place in civilian life, the nights spent feeling like he didn't belong anywhere. Tom listened, offering quiet words of encouragement, knowing that sometimes, just being there was enough.

By the end of the event, Tom felt a sense of fulfillment he hadn't expected. He'd spent so long feeling like he was the one in need of help, the one who had nothing to offer. But standing there, seeing the relief in Ben's eyes, he realized that he'd found something he hadn't known he was looking for a purpose beyond his own survival.

In the days that followed, Tom continued attending the support group, his connection with the other members deepening with each session. He and Julia had become close friends, their bond forged in shared struggles and quiet understanding. They'd started meeting outside of the group, grabbing coffee or going for walks, talking about everything from their favorite movies to their darkest fears.

One afternoon, as they sat on a bench overlooking the lake, Julia turned to him, her expression thoughtful. "You seem…different lately," she said, her voice soft. "Like you've found something to hold onto."

Tom looked out at the water, the reflection of the sky shimmering on the surface. "I think I have," he admitted. "Helping out at the event felt good. For the first time, I felt like I was more than just…damaged. Like I actually had something to give."

Julia smiled, a hint of pride in her expression. "You do, Tom. More than you realize. Sometimes, the people who've been through the worst are the ones who have the most to offer."

They sat in comfortable silence, the weight of her words settling over him. For so long, he'd thought of himself as broken, as someone who needed fixing. But now, he was beginning to see himself in a new light not as a victim of his circumstances, but as someone who could make a difference, even in small ways.

As the weeks went by, Tom found himself volunteering more, helping organize events and reaching out to other veterans in need. He'd started to become a familiar face at the community center, someone people could count on, someone they could turn to. He still had his struggles, his dark days and restless nights, but now, he had something to keep him going, a purpose that gave his life meaning.

One evening, after a long day of volunteering, he returned home, feeling a sense of contentment that was new, unfamiliar but welcome. His mother was waiting for him in the kitchen, a cup of tea in her hands, her face soft with a mixture of pride and relief.

"You've been busy lately," she said, her voice warm.

Tom nodded, a small smile tugging at his lips. "Yeah. Feels…good to stay busy. Feels like I'm doing something that matters."

She reached out, placing a hand on his arm, her eyes filled with gratitude. "We're proud of you, Tom. All of us. You've come a long way."

Her words sank into him, filling the empty spaces he hadn't known were there. He still had a long way to go, he knew that. But for the first time, he felt like he was on the right path, like he was building a life he could be proud of.

As he stood there, surrounded by the warmth of his home, he felt a sense of peace settle over him, a quiet strength that had been absent for so long. He wasn't healed, not yet, but he was healing. And that, he realized, was more than enough.

CHAPTER 8

NEW BEGINNINGS

Months had passed since Tom first walked into the veterans' support group, feeling like he didn't belong anywhere. Each week had brought its own small battles and victories, moments of doubt and strength. Now, as spring began to warm the town and new leaves unfolded on the trees, Tom felt a quiet sense of renewal in his own life, too.

He'd started working part-time at the community center, officially joining the veterans' outreach team. The job wasn't glamorous, and it didn't pay much, but it gave him purpose. He organized meetings, helped other veterans find resources, and spent hours simply listening to their stories. He was no longer just surviving; he was building something that mattered.

One Friday evening, Tom was helping set up for a monthly veterans' mixer event. It was a simple gathering with coffee, pastries, and a place for veterans to socialize and connect. His fellow group member Julia arrived early to help, and they worked side by side, arranging chairs and setting out refreshments.

As they worked, Julia glanced over at him with a smile. "You've really come a long way, you know that?"

Tom looked at her, surprised by the pride in her voice. "It's because of this place. And people like you. I don't know where I'd be without all of this."

She nodded, her expression thoughtful. "It's a team effort. We're all helping each other here. But you've given a lot back, Tom. You're making a difference."

The words filled him with a warmth he hadn't expected. For the first time in a long time, he felt at home—not just in the room, but in himself. It was a strange feeling, this sense of peace, but he welcomed it.

Later that evening, as the room filled with veterans and familiar faces, Tom noticed a man standing by the door, looking nervous and unsure. He was older, maybe in his 50s, with a hard expression that softened when he saw Tom approach.

"Hey there," Tom said, extending his hand. "I'm Tom. You new here?"

The man nodded, giving Tom's hand a firm shake. "Yeah. Name's Frank. I, uh…wasn't sure if this was the right place for me. But I heard about the event and figured I'd check it out."

Tom smiled, recognizing the hesitation, the guarded expression. "Well, you're in the right place, Frank. Trust me. I

felt the same way when I first came here. But these people…
they understand."

Frank nodded slowly, his shoulders relaxing a bit. As they
talked, Tom shared his own experiences, the struggles he'd
faced, and the support he'd found in the group. By the end of
the conversation, Frank was smiling, and Tom felt a familiar
sense of fulfillment—a reminder of why he'd chosen to stay
involved in the community center's work.

Throughout the evening, Tom watched as the veterans
mingled, talked, and laughed. The room was filled with a
kind of warmth, a sense of belonging that felt like a balm on
old wounds. Tom knew he couldn't erase the past, couldn't
undo the scars he carried, but here, in this room, he was
reminded that healing was possible.

The next day, Tom's family gathered at the house for
dinner, a small celebration of his six months of sobriety. His
mother had cooked his favorite meal, and Rachel had
brought a cake, complete with a slightly crooked
"Congratulations" scrawled in icing. It was a simple affair, but
it meant more to Tom than he could put into words.

As they sat around the table, laughing and sharing stories,
Tom felt a sense of contentment settle over him. He hadn't
realized how much he'd missed these moments, the ease of
being with family, of feeling connected to something solid
and real.

After dinner, his father pulled him aside, leading him out to the back porch. The night air was cool, and they stood in comfortable silence for a moment, looking out at the quiet street.

"I'm proud of you, Tom," his father said finally, his voice steady but filled with emotion. "I know we don't always say it, but…we've seen how hard you've worked. We've seen the changes. And it means the world to us."

Tom looked at his father, surprised by the raw honesty in his voice. For so long, he'd thought he was a disappointment, a burden his family had to bear. But now, hearing his father's words, he felt a sense of validation, a recognition of the journey he'd been on.

"Thanks, Dad," he replied, his voice thick with emotion. "I…couldn't have done it without you. All of you."

They stood there for a while, the silence filled with understanding, a bridge mending between them. At that moment, Tom realized that he'd found his way back, not just to his family, but to himself.

The next few weeks flew by, filled with work at the community center, moments spent with friends, and quiet evenings with his family. Tom's life was simple, but it was full, filled with connections and purpose that had once felt impossible. He knew he'd still face challenges, that some days would be harder than others. But now, he had a support system, people who cared, and a reason to keep going.

One Saturday morning, he joined Rachel on a hike, something they'd started doing regularly. As they climbed the trail, she looked over at him, a hint of mischief in her eyes.

"So, big brother, what's next for you? You seem…different lately. Like you've got plans."

Tom thought about it, feeling a spark of excitement mixed with uncertainty. "I don't know. I think I just want to keep helping people. Maybe even go back to school, get some training in counseling or something."

Rachel grinned, nudging his shoulder. "You'd be great at that, you know. People trust you, Tom. You've got a way of making them feel safe."

Her words warmed him, and he felt a sense of possibility unfurling inside him. He'd spent so long feeling lost, like he didn't have a future. But now, he saw a path forward, one that felt right, one that would let him continue the work he'd started.

As they finished their hike and returned to the trailhead, Tom looked out at the landscape, the sun casting a warm glow over the hills. He felt a sense of peace, a quiet acceptance of the journey he'd been on. He knew he'd never be the person he was before, that the scars he carried would always be a part of him. But now, those scars felt less like wounds and more like marks of resilience, reminders of the strength he'd found within himself.

In the months to come, Tom continued his work at the community center, eventually enrolling in classes to become a counselor. His days were filled with purpose, with the knowledge that he was helping others find their way, just as he had.

And in those quiet moments, sitting with a fellow veteran, listening to their story, he felt a sense of fulfillment he'd never known. He'd come full circle, finding healing not just for himself, but for those who needed it most.

CHAPTER 9

THE JOB SEARCH

Tom's days at the community center had brought him a sense of fulfillment he hadn't felt in a long time. Helping other veterans, listening to their stories, and giving them a sense of belonging, it felt like he was part of something larger than himself. But while his work at the center was rewarding, it wasn't a paid position, and he knew he couldn't live on volunteer work alone. He needed a real job, something that would give him both stability and a sense of independence.

His father had offered to help him find work with one of his contacts, but Tom had declined, wanting to do it on his own. He'd spent enough time depending on others, leaning on his family when he couldn't stand on his own. Now, he was determined to prove that he could build a life for himself.

For the next few weeks, Tom threw himself into the job search, applying for everything he could find: warehouse jobs, security positions, even some office work. He adjusted his resume, omitting details that hinted too strongly at his military past. He knew that some employers saw veterans as a risk, especially those with medical discharges. He'd experienced it before, the wary looks, the polite but dismissive rejections. But he didn't let it deter him. He'd come too far to let a few setbacks push him back into the darkness.

However, as the days turned into weeks and the rejections piled up, Tom's frustration began to grow. Each email, each phone call that ended in a rejection, felt like another blow to his confidence, another reminder of the gap between his past and the civilian world he was trying to reenter. He began to wonder if there was a place for him out here at all.

One afternoon, after a long day of sending applications, Tom sat in his truck outside a local office building, clutching his resume in his hand. He'd been here twice before, both times walking away after convincing himself he didn't belong. But today, he was determined to at least get through the door. Taking a deep breath, he got out of the truck and walked inside.

The receptionist greeted him politely, glancing at his resume before directing him to a small waiting area. Tom sat down, tapping his foot nervously, his mind racing with thoughts of all the ways this could go wrong. When the hiring manager finally called him in, Tom stood, smoothing his shirt and forcing a calm expression.

The manager, a middle-aged man named Frank with a no-nonsense demeanor, gestured for Tom to take a seat. He glanced over Tom's resume, his face impassive. "I see you served in the military," he said, his tone neutral.

"Yes, sir," Tom replied, keeping his voice steady. "I served in the Army for several years before my discharge."

Frank nodded, his gaze sharp. "And what brings you to us? This isn't exactly a military role."

Tom hesitated, choosing his words carefully. "I'm looking for a new start. I have experience with discipline, teamwork, and handling high-stress situations. I think those skills could be valuable here."

Frank leaned back, studying him. "Look, Tom, I appreciate your service. I really do. But...we're looking for someone with more civilian experience. This is a fast-paced environment, and we need someone who can hit the ground running."

Tom felt the familiar sting of rejection, the disappointment settling in his chest. He nodded, his voice tight. "I understand."

Frank sighed, his expression softening slightly. "Look, don't take this the wrong way. I know it's tough out there for veterans. But this kind of job... it's just different from what you're used to."

Tom forced a smile, thanking Frank for his time, even as he felt frustration simmering beneath the surface. As he walked out of the building, he could feel the weight of his failure pressing down on him, a reminder of how different his world had been from the one he was trying to join.

That evening, Tom sat on his front porch, nursing a glass of water as he watched the sun dip below the horizon. He'd spent years following orders, performing tasks with precision and purpose. But out here, he felt adrift, like a tool that no longer had a purpose.

The door creaked open behind him, and his mother stepped out, a concerned look in her eyes. "Rough day?" she asked, sitting beside him.

Tom nodded, staring down at the glass in his hands. "It's… harder than I thought it would be. I keep thinking I'm making progress, but then something like today happens, and it feels like I'm right back where I started."

His mother reached over, placing a hand on his shoulder. "You're not where you started, Tom. You've come a long way. And sometimes, finding the right path takes time. Don't let one bad day make you doubt everything."

Her words offered some comfort, but the frustration still lingered. He'd fought so hard to rebuild himself, to find a place in the world, and now it felt like he was back at square one. He knew he had skills, discipline, and the drive to succeed, but none of that seemed to matter out here.

Over the next few days, Tom kept applying, each rejection hitting him a little harder, each polite "We'll keep your resume on file" feeling like a slap in the face. His self-doubt began to creep back in, the familiar voice telling him he was unfit, that he'd never belong. He started missing a few group meetings, too embarrassed to share his struggles with the others. He felt like a failure, like he was letting everyone down.

But one evening, as he sat in his room staring blankly at yet another rejection email, he heard his phone buzz. It was a text from Julia, a simple message that read, Haven't seen you at group. Miss having you there.

Tom stared at the message, feeling a flicker of something close to relief. He hadn't realized how much he'd isolated himself, how much he'd let his disappointment pull him back into the shadows. Julia's message reminded him that he wasn't alone, that he had people who understood, who wouldn't judge him for struggling.

Taking a deep breath, he replied, I'll be there next time. Thanks.

At the next group meeting, Tom shared his experiences, the difficulty of finding work, the constant rejections. The others listened without judgment, nodding in understanding. Julia spoke up, sharing her own struggles with job hunting, the countless times she'd felt overlooked because of her background.

Carl, the group leader, offered a few words of encouragement. "This process isn't easy, Tom. But you've got resilience. You've faced things most people can't even imagine. The right place will see that, and they'll value what you bring."

Tom left the meeting that night feeling a renewed sense of determination. He knew the road ahead would still be difficult, that he'd face more setbacks. But he was reminded that he wasn't alone, that he had a community of people who believed in him, even when he struggled to believe in himself.

In the weeks that followed, Tom kept applying, each rejection becoming a little easier to bear. He kept attending the group meetings, finding strength in the support and encouragement of his fellow veterans. And finally, one morning, he received a call from the community center offering him a full-time position as a veterans' liaison, a role that would allow him to continue his work with other veterans, providing resources and support to those in need.

As he hung up the phone, a sense of relief washed over him. It wasn't the job he'd originally imagined, but it was one that felt meaningful, one that allowed him to use his experiences to help others. He'd found his place, his purpose, and it was one he could truly be proud of.

He'd finally found his footing in the civilian world, and while the road had been rough, he knew he was exactly where he needed to be.

CHAPTER 10

ANOTHER LIFE

A few weeks into his new position at the community center, Tom had settled into a routine that brought him a quiet sense of satisfaction. The days were full but purposeful, and each time he helped another veteran navigate resources or connect with support, he felt a bit more at home in his role. Life was far from perfect, but he was beginning to see a future for himself that didn't feel weighed down by the past.

One Saturday afternoon, Tom was running errands in town when he saw her. Sarah, standing outside a coffee shop, looking just as he remembered, maybe a bit older, a bit more mature, but still with the same warm, genuine smile. His heart tightened as he watched her laugh, her head tilting slightly as she listened to the man beside her, who was holding the hand of a little girl with curly brown hair.

For a moment, Tom thought about turning around, walking the other way before she noticed him. But just as he made the decision, she glanced his way, her eyes widening in recognition. A mixture of surprise and warmth filled her face, and before he knew it, she was walking toward him.

"Tom?" she asked, her voice tinged with disbelief. "It's been so long."

Tom managed a small smile, his voice a bit stiff. "Hey, Sarah. Yeah, it's… been a while."

She gestured to the man and the little girl, who had moved into the coffee shop, giving them space. "That's my husband, Josh, and our daughter, Lila," she said, her tone both proud and soft. "I've heard you're back in town, but I wasn't sure if I'd ever run into you."

Tom nodded, swallowing against the sudden tightness in his throat. Seeing Sarah with her family stirred emotions he hadn't expected, a blend of happiness for her and a lingering ache for what might have been. "Yeah, I'm back," he replied. "Been here a few months, actually. Trying to…figure things out."

She looked at him, her eyes filled with a kindness he'd almost forgotten. "I'm really glad you're back, Tom. I know it wasn't easy for you, coming home. I've thought about you a lot, and wondered how you were doing."

They stood in silence for a moment, the weight of unsaid things hanging between them. Tom remembered the last time he'd seen her, the night before he left for his last deployment. They'd had a quiet dinner together, filled with promises to keep in touch, to pick things up when he came back. But after his return, broken and distant, he'd pushed her away, too ashamed and too lost to let her in. Eventually, he'd let her go, convinced she deserved someone who could offer her the life she wanted.

Now, standing here, he realized that part of him had never fully let go of the guilt, the sense of regret that lingered whenever he thought of her. She'd moved on, found happiness, but he hadn't been there for her the way he'd promised.

"So, what about you?" she asked, breaking the silence. "How have you been?"

Tom hesitated, unsure how to answer. "It's been… a journey," he admitted. "I'm working at the community center now, helping other veterans. It's… good. Keeps me focused."

She nodded, her smile genuine. "That's wonderful, Tom. I always knew you'd find a way to make a difference."

He chuckled, a bit self-conscious. "I don't know if I'm making much of a difference, but… it feels good to be doing something meaningful."

They continued talking for a few more minutes, catching up on the small details of their lives. Tom found himself relaxing, the old connection between them resurfacing, though now it felt softer, gentler a friendship built on mutual respect and shared history rather than romance.

Finally, Sarah glanced back toward the coffee shop, where her husband and daughter were waiting. "I should get back to them," she said, a hint of reluctance in her voice. "But I'm really glad we ran into each other. And I'm so proud of you, Tom. I hope you know that."

He smiled, feeling a warmth in her words that soothed some of the old wounds he'd carried. "Thank you, Sarah. I'm...happy for you. You deserve all of this."

As they said their goodbyes, Tom watched her walk back to her family, a bittersweet feeling settling over him. Seeing Sarah with her husband and daughter brought a sense of closure, a recognition that he'd made the right choice by letting her go. She'd found happiness, and he was genuinely glad for her. For the first time, he felt at peace with the decision, knowing that she was exactly where she was meant to be.

That evening, as Tom sat on his porch, he thought about the life he'd left behind, the person he'd been before the army. Meeting Sarah again had reminded him of how much he'd changed, how far he'd come. He'd let go of a lot of things, dreams, relationships, pieces of himself he'd never get back. But he was beginning to accept that he wasn't the same person, and that was okay.

He'd spent so long mourning the life he thought he'd have that he'd almost forgotten the one he was building now. He didn't have a family of his own, didn't have the stability he'd once imagined. But he had purpose, community, and a growing sense of inner strength.

As he sat in the quiet, he thought about reaching out to Julia, his friend from the support group. She'd been a steady presence in his life, someone who understood his journey without needing explanations. He wasn't sure what he felt for her was friendship or something deeper but he knew she was important to him, that she'd become someone he relied on.

Without overthinking, he picked up his phone and sent her a message: Hey, just wanted to say thanks for being there. I know I don't always say it, but it means a lot.

Her reply came a few minutes later: Anytime, Tom. You're not getting rid of me that easily. Let's grab coffee soon?

He smiled, feeling a sense of gratitude he hadn't felt in a long time. His past would always be a part of him, but he was learning that it didn't have to define him. He had friends, family, and a purpose. And maybe, just maybe, he could find happiness in this life, in this version of himself.

CHAPTER 11

NEW CONNECTIONS

Tom's work at the community center had grown to feel like a second home. The long days were filled with purpose, and each time he saw a veteran walk out the door with a sense of relief or hope, he felt the quiet satisfaction of knowing he'd helped in some way. But despite the sense of accomplishment, one person stayed on his mind more than the others: Ben, the young veteran he'd met at the outreach event.

Ben had started attending the support group regularly, his guarded demeanor gradually softening as he became more comfortable. He was quiet, often sitting at the edge of the circle, but Tom noticed him watching, listening, taking in every word. They hadn't spoken much outside of group discussions, but Tom felt a connection with him, a silent understanding. Ben reminded him of himself—not just because of their shared experiences but because of the way Ben struggled to let others in, the way he carried himself like he was holding the weight of the world on his shoulders.

One afternoon, after a particularly heavy group session, Tom caught up with Ben as he was leaving the community center. "Hey, you got a few minutes?" he asked, keeping his tone casual.

Ben shrugged, his hands stuffed into his pockets. "Sure. What's up?"

"Thought maybe we could grab a coffee," Tom suggested. "Figured it might be nice to talk outside of the group."

Ben hesitated, his expression guarded, but then he nodded. "Yeah. Alright. I guess I could go for a coffee."

They walked to a small café down the street, the silence between them comfortable but filled with an unspoken tension. Tom ordered their drinks, and they took a seat by the window. For a few minutes, neither of them spoke, and Tom could tell Ben was wrestling with something, debating whether or not to let his guard down.

Finally, Ben broke the silence. "So… why are you doing this?"

Tom looked at him, surprised by the blunt question. "Doing what?"

Ben glanced down, fidgeting with his cup. "Helping out. Talking to me. I know a lot of people don't…get it."

Tom nodded slowly, understanding the uncertainty behind Ben's words. "I get it more than you might think," he replied. "When I first came back, I thought I had to handle everything on my own. Thought maybe no one would understand what

I'd been through. But I've learned that sometimes, the best way to find peace is to help others find it too."

Ben looked away, his jaw tightening. "It's just… hard. I thought coming back would be easy, you know? Like, I'd just pick up where I left off. But it's not like that. Nothing feels… right."

Tom nodded, his heart aching with empathy. "Yeah. It's not easy. But you don't have to do it alone, Ben. I tried that, and it only made things worse. I don't have all the answers, but I do know that talking to people who get it makes a difference."

Ben took a deep breath, his gaze distant. "Sometimes it feels like everything's… too much. Like I can't breathe. And I keep thinking… what if this never goes away?"

Tom's chest tightened at the raw honesty in Ben's voice. He'd been there, in that same place, feeling like there was no way out. "I won't lie to you," he said quietly. "It doesn't just… go away. But it does get easier. You learn to carry it, to live with it without letting it control you. But that takes time, and it takes people. People who understand."

Ben nodded slowly, his eyes filled with a vulnerability he'd been hiding. "I just don't know if I can do it."

"You can," Tom said, his voice steady. "You're already doing it. Showing up, talking to people, letting yourself be honest about how you feel and that's the hardest part. But you're doing it."

They sat in silence for a few moments, the weight of Ben's words settling between them. Tom felt a surge of pride, a sense of purpose in being there for Ben. It was a reminder of his own journey, of how far he'd come, and of the strength he'd found along the way.

As they finished their coffee, Ben looked at him, a hint of gratitude in his expression. "Thanks, Tom. I know I don't say much, but… this helps."

Tom smiled, clapping him on the shoulder. "Anytime, Ben. You're not alone in this."

Over the following weeks, Tom and Ben grew closer, meeting for coffee regularly and talking about everything from their military experiences to their struggles adjusting to civilian life. Tom saw a bit of himself in Ben's guarded nature, his reluctance to trust others, and he was reminded of the support he'd received from people like Carl and Julia, who had been there for him when he was at his lowest.

One evening, as they walked together after a group meeting, Ben paused, looking at Tom with a serious expression. "I don't know if I could've made it this far without you," he admitted. "It feels like… I've finally got someone who gets it."

Tom felt a swell of pride and gratitude. He'd been lost once, too, struggling to find his place in the world. But helping Ben, seeing him grow stronger and more confident, had given Tom a new sense of purpose. He wasn't just surviving anymore; he was helping others do the same.

"Anytime, Ben," he said, his voice filled with sincerity. "We're in this together."

Ben nodded, his face softening. "I think… I think I might be ready to look for work again. Maybe even go back to school. I mean, it's a long shot, but… I've got to try."

Tom clapped him on the back, feeling a rush of excitement. "That's amazing, Ben. You've got what it takes. I know it."

They walked in silence, the weight of their shared journey settling over them. Tom realized that helping Ben had healed parts of himself he hadn't known were still broken. It was a reminder that his own path to recovery was ongoing, but it was no longer a lonely one. He had friends, a purpose, and a growing confidence that he was exactly where he needed to be.

That night, Tom returned home with a sense of peace. He'd spent so long thinking he had nothing left to give, but now he saw that wasn't true. He'd become a guide, a mentor, someone who could offer hope to those who were struggling. In helping Ben, he'd found healing for himself, a reminder of his own resilience and strength.

For the first time in a long time, he felt truly at home in his life, surrounded by people who understood him, who valued him not just for his past, but for who he was now. And he knew, deep down, that he was finally on the right path, a path that he would continue to walk. Not only just for himself, but for others who needed him too.

CHAPTER 12

FAMILY BONDS

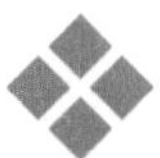

The following Sunday, Tom found himself sitting in his parents' living room, surrounded by family. His mother had organized a small gathering, an excuse for everyone to come together for a simple meal and some time spent catching up. Tom had initially felt hesitant about coming, but he'd noticed that each time he visited, the sense of tension in his family's eyes seemed to soften.

Rachel had driven up for the weekend, and she sat across from him, her face lit with excitement as she recounted a funny story from her work. Tom found himself laughing along, feeling more relaxed than he'd been in a long time. As he looked around the room, he realized how much he'd missed these moments the simplicity of being together, the warmth of shared laughter.

After dinner, Rachel pulled him aside, leading him to the backyard where they could talk in private. The night air was cool, and they sat on the porch steps, a comfortable silence settling between them.

Rachel looked over at him, her expression serious but filled with affection. "You seem… different, Tom. Like you're finally finding your place."

Tom nodded, glancing out at the stars. "Yeah, I think I am. For the first time, I feel like I have a purpose, like I'm doing something that matters."

She reached over, giving his hand a gentle squeeze. "I'm proud of you, you know. I've watched you struggle, and it broke my heart to see you go through all of that. But seeing you now… it feels like you're finally healing."

Tom swallowed, his throat tight with emotion. He'd never talked much about his experiences in the military or his struggles after coming home. It was easier to keep it all inside, to let his family think he was just "working things out." But he knew now that keeping them in the dark had only deepened the rift between them.

"Rach, there's…a lot I've kept from you," he admitted, his voice barely above a whisper. "I thought I was protecting you by not talking about it. But I realize now that shutting you all out wasn't fair. I went through some dark times, and I didn't know how to deal with it. I still don't, sometimes."

Rachel looked at him, her eyes filled with understanding. "I get it, Tom. I really do. But you don't have to carry this alone. We're your family. We're here for you, no matter what."

The sincerity in her voice brought a wave of relief, a sense of comfort that he hadn't realized he was missing. He'd spent so long thinking he had to protect his family from his pain, but now, he saw that they wanted to share the burden, to be a part of his journey.

"I want to be better, Rach," he said quietly. "Not just for me, but for you, Mom, and Dad. I know I haven't been easy to be around, and I'm sorry for that."

She wrapped her arms around him in a tight hug, her voice filled with warmth. "You don't have to apologize, Tom. We love you, and we're just glad to see you finding your way."

They sat in silence for a few moments, the weight of unspoken words settling between them. Tom felt a sense of closeness he hadn't felt in years, a reminder that he was part of something bigger than himself, a family that loved him no matter what.

Over the next few weeks, Tom continued to spend more time with his family, gradually opening up about his journey, sharing bits and pieces of his struggles. His parents listened without judgment, their presence a steady comfort that grounded him. For so long, he'd thought they wouldn't understand, that his pain was something he had to face alone. But now, he saw that letting them in, allowing them to see the parts of himself he'd hidden, was part of his healing.

One evening, as he sat with his father in the living room, his dad looked over at him, his face filled with a rare vulnerability. "Tom, I just want you to know that… I'm proud of you. I know I don't always say it, but I am. You've been through so much, and seeing the man you're becoming… it means the world to me."

Tom felt a lump rise in his throat, the words hitting him in a way he hadn't expected. He'd always thought his father was disappointed in him, that he'd let him down by coming back so broken. But now, hearing his father's pride and love, he felt a weight lift from his shoulders, a sense of acceptance that soothed old wounds.

"Thanks, Dad," he said, his voice thick with emotion. "I wouldn't have made it this far without you, without all of you. I know I didn't make it easy."

His father reached over, giving his shoulder a firm squeeze. "You don't have to carry everything on your own, Tom. We're here for you, always."

As they sat together in the quiet, Tom realized that his family had become a pillar of strength, a source of support he hadn't allowed himself to lean on before. He'd always thought he had to face his battles alone, but now, he saw that he was part of something larger, a network of love and understanding that would be there through every challenge.

One weekend, Rachel suggested they go hiking together, an activity they'd loved before Tom left for the military. They packed their bags and drove out to a trail they'd hiked countless times as kids. The walk was peaceful, the familiar sights and sounds grounding Tom in a way that felt both nostalgic and comforting.

As they reached a viewpoint overlooking the valley, Rachel looked at him, a soft smile on her face. "I'm really glad you're home, Tom. It feels like…like I have my big brother back."

Tom smiled, feeling a sense of gratitude that ran deep. "I'm glad, too, Rach. I missed this. I missed us."

They sat in silence, watching the sun dip below the horizon, the sky painted in shades of pink and orange. In that moment, Tom felt a sense of peace, a quiet acceptance that he hadn't felt in a long time. He knew he still had a long way to go, that the road to healing was far from over. But now, he had his family by his side, and that made all the difference.

For so long, he'd thought he was broken beyond repair, that his family would never understand the weight he carried. But now, he saw that they were part of his journey, part of the strength he needed to move forward. They'd become his anchor, his reminder that he was never truly alone.

As they hiked back down, Rachel's laughter echoing in the cool evening air, Tom felt a renewed sense of purpose, a quiet confidence that he was exactly where he needed to be. He was finding his way, one step at a time, with the people who mattered most by his side.

CHAPTER 13

HONORING THE FALLEN

Tom had been attending the veterans' support group for nearly a year now, and each session brought him closer to the people who'd become his community. He'd developed friendships that felt like lifelines, bonds that grounded him in ways he hadn't felt since he left the military. One of those friendships was with Charlie, the older veteran who'd been a mentor to him since his first days at the community center.

One evening after a meeting, as they were closing up the room, Charlie approached Tom with a thoughtful look. "Got a minute, kid?" he asked, his voice gruff but warm.

"Of course, what's up?" Tom replied, glancing over as he stacked the last of the chairs.

Charlie looked down, fiddling with his watch, his expression shifting to something more somber. "There's an event coming up next weekend, an annual remembrance ceremony for fallen soldiers. A lot of the guys from our unit usually go. It's a way to honor those we lost, to remember them together." He paused, meeting Tom's eyes. "I thought maybe you'd like to join me."

Tom felt his chest tighten, a mixture of emotions flooding him all at once pride, sadness, and a deep-seated fear he couldn't quite name. He hadn't been to any kind of memorial service since his return, and hadn't allowed himself to revisit those memories in any formal way. But the thought of honoring his fallen friends, of standing beside Charlie and other veterans who understood that loss, felt strangely comforting.

"Yeah," Tom said quietly, nodding. "I'd like that."

Charlie smiled, clapping him on the shoulder. "Good. It's not easy, but it's worth it. They deserve to be remembered."

The morning of the ceremony dawned cold and clear, the early light casting a soft glow over the cemetery where the service was held. Tom arrived early, feeling a knot of tension in his stomach as he took in the rows of white headstones stretching out before him. He hadn't been to a place like this since his return, and the weight of it all felt like a physical presence, pressing down on him.

Charlie arrived shortly after, and they walked to the gathering area together in silence. Veterans of all ages stood quietly, some holding flags, others clutching flowers or photos. The air was filled with a solemn reverence, a collective grief that felt both heavy and shared. Tom took a deep breath, steadying himself, feeling the weight of his own memories pressing against the present.

As the ceremony began, the speakers took turns sharing stories of the fallen, memories of friendship, of courage, of sacrifice. Tom listened, his mind drifting back to his own memories, the faces of friends he'd lost and names he still carried in his heart. He felt the familiar ache of guilt, the weight of survivor's remorse that had followed him since his discharge. But standing there among others who understood that pain, he felt a quiet strength, a reminder that he wasn't alone in carrying that weight.

When it came time for Charlie to speak, Tom watched as his friend stepped forward, his voice steady but filled with emotion. Charlie shared a story about a fellow soldier from their unit, a friend who'd always been the first to volunteer, the one who'd made them all laugh even in the darkest moments.

"He didn't make it home," Charlie said, his voice catching slightly. "But he lives on in each of us. In every story we tell, every time we gather like this. He's here with us."

As Charlie spoke, Tom felt tears prick his eyes, his chest tightening as he allowed himself to feel the grief he'd kept locked away. For so long, he'd been afraid to confront that pain, to acknowledge the loss of those he'd fought beside. But here, among those who understood, he felt a sense of release, a permission to grieve.

After the ceremony, Charlie led Tom to a quiet spot beneath a large oak tree, where they could sit in the shade.

For a while, they didn't speak, each lost in his own thoughts, the weight of the ceremony settling over them.

Finally, Charlie broke the silence, his voice low. "I know it's not easy remembering them like this. But it's important. We carry their memory because they can't. And that's how we honor them."

Tom nodded, his throat tight. "I've spent so long trying to forget, to push it all down. But being here… it feels like the right thing. Like I can finally let myself remember them without…without falling apart."

Charlie looked at him, his gaze steady. "That's because you're stronger than you think, kid. We're all broken in some way, but that doesn't mean we're weak. It means we've lived through something. And those memories, those people they're part of us. You don't have to carry them alone."

Tom felt a surge of gratitude, a warmth that pushed back against the cold ache of loss. For so long, he'd thought of his memories as a burden, something to be hidden away. But now, he saw them as something else, a part of his story, a reminder of the friendships, the sacrifices, the bonds that had shaped him.

"Thank you, Charlie," he said quietly. "For everything."

Charlie smiled, clapping him on the back. "Anytime. We're in this together, all of us. And don't you forget it."

That evening, Tom returned home with a sense of peace he hadn't expected. The ceremony had been painful, but it had also brought a sense of closure, a release from the weight of guilt and regret he'd carried for so long. He realized now that honoring his friends didn't mean he had to be trapped by their memory. Instead, he could carry them with him, allowing their legacy to become a part of his life rather than a burden.

As he sat on his porch, watching the stars, he thought about the people he'd lost, the sacrifices they'd made. He knew that they'd want him to live, to find happiness, to make the most of the life he'd been given. And for the first time, he felt like he could honor that wish not by forgetting, but by embracing the life he was building.

He felt a sense of acceptance settle over him, a quiet understanding that he didn't have to face his memories alone. He had his family, his friends, and the veterans who stood beside him at the ceremony. Together, they carried the memory of those who hadn't made it home, a collective strength that was greater than any one person's burden.

In the quiet of the night, Tom whispered a silent promise to his fallen friends, a promise to live fully, to honor their memory by finding joy, by helping others, by continuing the journey they'd begun together. He knew that the road ahead would still have its challenges, but he was no longer afraid. He was stronger than he'd ever known, and he was ready to move forward, carrying both his memories and his hope into the future.

CHAPTER 14

A NEW LIFE

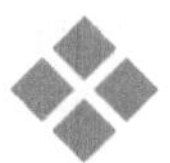

In the months following the ceremony, Tom felt a shift within himself, a quiet but steady confidence he hadn't known in years. He'd been at the community center for nearly a year now, his role growing as he took on more responsibilities. Carl had even given him the title of Veterans' Program Coordinator, a position that allowed him to oversee outreach efforts, lead meetings, and organize events for veterans in need. The work was demanding but fulfilling, each day giving him a renewed sense of purpose.

Tom's days were now filled with a busy rhythm that he relished. He helped other veterans navigate resources, organized support groups, and planned events to foster connection and community. For the first time, he felt rooted, secure in the knowledge that he was making a difference. His past had given him insight and empathy, allowing him to connect with those he helped on a level few could understand.

One Friday afternoon, Carl stopped by his office, leaning against the doorframe with a smile. "How's it going in here, Mr. Coordinator?"

Tom looked up from his stack of paperwork, grinning. "Busy, but good. Never thought I'd be sitting behind a desk, organizing events. Feels…surreal sometimes."

Carl chuckled, crossing his arms. "You're a natural, Tom. I knew from the moment you started coming to the group that you had something special: a way of connecting with people, making them feel safe. That's a rare gift."

Tom felt a warmth spread through him, a quiet pride that he'd never fully allowed himself to feel. "Thanks, Carl. It means a lot, coming from you. I just… I want to give back. To help others the way you and the group helped me."

Carl nodded, his expression thoughtful. "You're doing just that. And I'm proud of you, kid. You've come a long way."

After Carl left, Tom sat for a moment, letting the words sink in. He realized that he hadn't only found purpose here he'd found a family, a community of people who understood him in ways he hadn't thought possible. His role at the center was more than just a job; it was a calling, one that allowed him to live in honor of the friends he'd lost, to give back in a way that felt meaningful and real.

The next week, Tom organized an event for veterans and their families, a day of workshops, games, and a BBQ in the park. It was the biggest event he'd planned so far, and he'd poured hours into making sure every detail was perfect. He wanted to create a space where families could come together, where veterans could feel a sense of belonging and joy, even if just for a day.

As the event kicked off, Tom felt a surge of excitement mixed with nerves. Families trickled in, children laughing as they ran across the grass, veterans greeting each other with handshakes and hugs. The air was filled with a sense of warmth and camaraderie, a reminder of the community he'd helped build.

Throughout the day, Tom moved between groups, checking in with families, sharing stories, and helping with activities. He watched as veterans connected with each other, their laughter and stories filling the park, a contrast to the somber gatherings he'd attended in the past. This event wasn't about grief; it was about life, about celebrating the strength and resilience of those who'd served.

At one point, he spotted Ben sitting with his mother, a rare smile on his face. Ben caught Tom's eye and gave him a thumbs-up, mouthing, "Nice job." Tom grinned, feeling a surge of pride. Seeing Ben happy, seeing him surrounded by people who cared, reminded Tom of how far they'd both come. They'd both found their place in this community, and that shared journey had strengthened their bond.

Julia arrived a bit later, joining him as he helped set up the BBQ station. She'd been a steady presence in his life, her friendship a source of strength and comfort. They worked side by side, exchanging jokes as they flipped burgers and handed out plates.

As they served the food, Julia looked at him, her eyes filled with admiration. "You did an amazing job, Tom. This whole event... it's exactly what this community needed."

Tom smiled, a bit self-conscious. "I just wanted to give people a chance to come together, to feel...whole."

She reached out, giving his hand a squeeze. "You're doing more than that. You're giving people hope, a place to belong. That's something truly special."

They stood in silence for a moment, the weight of her words settling over him. For so long, he'd thought of himself as broken, as someone who needed saving. But now, he saw himself in a new light not as a victim of his past, but as someone who could make a difference, who could offer others the same support he'd found.

As the event wound down, Tom took a moment to stand back and take it all in. The park was filled with families and friends, laughter and conversation weaving through the warm evening air. He felt a sense of fulfillment, a quiet pride in knowing he'd helped create this moment, this place of healing and connection.

Carl approached him, clapping a hand on his shoulder. "Look at this, Tom. Look at what you've built."

Tom nodded, his eyes scanning the crowd. "It's not just me. It's all of us, the whole community. I just... helped bring everyone together."

Carl smiled, his gaze filled with pride. "That's what a leader does, kid. You've become someone people can look up to, someone they can trust. That's no small thing."

Tom felt the truth of Carl's words, a quiet acceptance settling over him. He'd spent so long searching for his purpose, for a reason to keep going. But now, he realized he'd found it not just in helping others, but in creating a space where people could feel seen, heard, and valued.

As the sun set over the park, casting a warm glow over the gathering, Tom felt a deep sense of peace. He knew he'd never forget the past, that his memories would always be a part of him. But now, those memories felt like pieces of a larger story, a reminder of the journey that had brought him here.

He was no longer defined by his pain, his loss, or his struggles. He was defined by his resilience, his compassion, and his commitment to helping others find their way. And in that, he'd found a new life, a life he could be proud of.

CHAPTER 15

A YEAR OF SOBRIETY

Tom had known the anniversary was coming up for a while, but it wasn't until the morning of, that he truly grasped the significance. One year! Three hundred and sixty-five days without a drink. It felt both monumental and surreal, a milestone that marked a journey from his darkest days to the steady, fulfilling life he was living now.

He woke up that morning with a quiet sense of pride, a feeling he hadn't allowed himself to fully embrace until now. He'd spent so much of the past year focusing on small steps, on surviving one day at a time, that he hadn't realized just how far he'd come. But now, as he sat on the edge of his bed, looking out at the morning light filtering through his window, he felt the weight of that year, the struggle, the growth, the resilience he'd built with each passing day.

His family had planned a small gathering at the community center to mark the occasion, a celebration of his one-year sobriety. It was a quiet event, meant for close friends, family, and a few members of his support group. Tom was both excited and nervous, the thought of being at the center of attention feeling both humbling and a bit overwhelming.

When he arrived at the community center that evening, he was met by a wave of warmth and familiar faces. His parents were there, beaming with pride, and Rachel stood beside them, her eyes shining with a mix of excitement and emotion. Carl and Julia were there as well, along with several members of the support group who had walked with him through the ups and downs of the past year.

As he stepped into the room, Carl clapped him on the back, grinning. "One year, Tom. That's no small feat. You should be proud."

Tom smiled, feeling a rush of gratitude. "Thanks, Carl. I couldn't have done it without all of you."

Carl nodded, his expression filled with warmth. "We're here because you showed up for yourself. Remember that. This journey you've earned every step."

The evening was filled with laughter, stories, and moments of reflection. Julia pulled him aside at one point, handing him a small card. "Just a little something," she said, smiling. "A reminder of how far you've come."

He opened the card to find a simple message: Strength is built in the quiet moments, one day at a time. Proud of you. Her words touched him deeply, a reminder of the countless moments of support she'd offered him along the way. She'd been a constant presence, someone who believed in him even when he struggled to believe in himself.

"Thank you," he said, his voice thick with emotion. "For everything."

She gave him a quick hug, a warm embrace that spoke volumes. "Always, Tom. You're not getting rid of me."

As the evening went on, Carl invited Tom to say a few words. Tom felt a pang of nerves as he stood up, looking out at the faces that had become his community, his family. He cleared his throat, taking a deep breath before he began.

"I never thought I'd be standing here today," he said, his voice steady but filled with emotion. "A year ago, I didn't think I had anything left to give. I was lost, angry, and convinced that my life had no purpose. But because of all of you, because of the support and love I found here, I was able to rebuild myself, one day at a time."

He paused, looking over at his parents, who were listening with proud, tearful expressions. "I've learned that healing isn't something you do alone. It's something you do with the people who stand by you, who remind you that you're worth fighting for. And because of all of you, I've found something I didn't think I'd ever have again... a sense of peace."

He took a deep breath, his heart swelling with gratitude. "This past year has been hard, but it's also been the most meaningful journey of my life. I know I still have a long way to go, but now, I'm not afraid of the road ahead. Thank you all for being part of this journey with me."

The room erupted in applause, and Tom felt a rush of warmth as he sat back down, his heart pounding with a mixture of pride and humility. He realized in that moment that he'd not only found his place in the world but had also become someone others could look to, someone who'd faced darkness and come through the other side.

After the celebration wound down, Tom lingered with his family, savoring the quiet moments together. Rachel hugged him tightly, her voice filled with emotion. "You're amazing, Tom. I hope you know that."

He chuckled, feeling a bit embarrassed but deeply grateful. "I'm just... trying to keep going, one day at a time."

His mother took his hand, her eyes filled with pride. "You're more than that, Tom. You're an inspiration to all of us."

His father, who was usually reserved, placed a firm hand on his shoulder. "You've shown us what true strength looks like, son. We're so proud of you."

The words settled over him, filling the empty spaces he hadn't known were there. For so long, he'd thought he was defined by his past, by his struggles. But now, he saw himself as someone stronger, someone who'd faced his own demons and found a way to keep going.

As they said their goodbyes and headed home, Tom felt a sense of peace that ran deep. He knew the journey wasn't over, that there would still be challenges ahead. But he was no longer afraid. He had a community, a purpose, and a family who believed in him. And, most importantly, he'd learned to believe in himself.

That night, as he lay in bed, he thought back over the past year the nights of doubt, the hard-won victories, the moments of connection that had carried him forward. He felt a profound sense of gratitude, a quiet acceptance of his journey and the person he'd become.

For the first time, he felt whole. Not because his pain had vanished or because he'd found all the answers, but because he'd learned to carry his past without letting it define him. He'd found a way to honor his memories, to live in a way that reflected his own resilience and the sacrifices of those he'd lost.

With a sense of calm, he closed his eyes, letting the weight of the past year settle over him. He was no longer just surviving, he was living, fully and completely, and he was ready to embrace whatever came next.

EPILOGUE

A QUIET PEACE

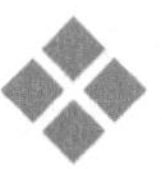

Years later, Tom stood outside the community center, looking up at the familiar building that had been his sanctuary, his lifeline, and eventually, his place of purpose. He was no longer the lost man who had walked through those doors looking for answers. Now, he was a part of something larger, a mentor, a friend, and a guide for veterans who, like him, were seeking a way to move forward.

The center had grown over the years, expanding to offer new programs, workshops, and counseling services. Tom had been there through each step of its evolution, helping to shape the space into a place where veterans and their families could find not just support but a sense of belonging. He'd seen countless men and women walk through those doors, burdened by the weight of their own memories, searching for hope. And each time he helped someone find their way, he felt a renewed sense of purpose, a quiet fulfillment that words couldn't quite capture.

As he walked inside, the familiar hum of voices filled the air, a comforting reminder of the community he'd helped build. He passed by rooms filled with people, some in quiet counseling sessions, others gathered in small groups, sharing stories and laughter. The walls were lined with photographs, memories of events and gatherings, each one a testament to the bonds formed and the healing shared within these walls.

Tom made his way to a small room at the end of the hall, where a group of new veterans was gathered, waiting for the start of their first support session. He paused at the doorway, looking at their faces, some filled with quiet hope, others marked by the same guarded expressions he'd once worn himself. He knew the struggles they carried, the uncertainty, the pain, and he understood the courage it took just to be here.

Taking a deep breath, he stepped inside, offering a warm smile as he introduced himself. "Welcome, everyone. My name's Tom, and I'm here to help you find your way. I know this isn't easy, but you're not alone. This place, this community, it's here for you, just like it was here for me."

As he began to speak, sharing his own story and the journey he'd taken, he felt the familiar weight of his past settle over him. But it was no longer a burden; it was a source of strength, a reminder of the resilience he'd built and the purpose he'd found. He was no longer defined by his pain, his losses, or his struggles. He was defined by the life he'd chosen to build, by the people he'd helped, and by the quiet peace he'd found in honoring his past.

After the session ended, Tom lingered in the room, watching as the veterans exchanged words, small smiles, and nods of understanding. He saw himself in their faces, in the tentative connections forming, in the slow unfolding of trust. This was what he'd dedicated his life. Creating a space where people could heal, where they could find the strength to keep going, even in the face of their darkest moments.

Later that evening, as he left the center and walked out into the crisp night air, he paused, looking up at the stars. He thought of the friends he'd lost, the memories that had once haunted him, and the people who had been there for him when he'd needed them most. He whispered a silent thank-you, a promise to continue living fully, to carry their memory with him, not as a weight but as a part of who he was.

In the years since his journey had begun, he'd learned that healing wasn't a destination but a lifelong path, one that required courage, patience, and the willingness to keep moving forward. He'd come to understand that peace wasn't something he could find in isolation but something he could build, moment by moment, with the people who'd chosen to walk beside him.

As he stood there, surrounded by the quiet of the night, he felt a deep sense of gratitude. A gratitude for his family, for his friends, for the veterans who had become his community, and for the life he'd fought to build. He knew he'd never forget the pain, the losses, the struggles that had shaped him. But he also knew that he'd found something more powerful. A life filled with purpose, resilience, and quiet peace.

With a final look at the stars, Tom turned and walked toward his car, his steps steady, his heart full. He was exactly where and who he needed to be.

REMEMBER IF YOU EVER THINK YOU ARE ALONE YOU ARE NOT! THESE NUMBERS AND EMAILS ARE HERE TO HELP EVERYONE!!

Immediate Crisis Support:

- **988 Suicide & Crisis Lifeline:** A nationwide service offering free, confidential support 24/7 for individuals in distress.
  - Call or Text: 988
  - **Chat Online:** <u>988lifeline.org</u>
  - This lifeline connects callers to trained counselors who provide support for mental health crises, including substance use issues.

Veteran-Specific Resources:

- **Veterans Crisis Line:** Dedicated to veterans in crisis, providing confidential assistance 24/7.
  - **Call:** 988 and press 1
  - **Text:** 838255
  - **Chat Online:** <u>veteranscrisisline.net</u>
  - This service connects veterans with qualified responders, many of whom are veterans themselves.

- **VA Substance Use Disorder Treatment:** The Department of Veterans Affairs offers comprehensive treatment programs for veterans dealing with substance use issues.
  - **Information:** <u>va.gov/health-care/health-needs-conditions/substance-use-problems/</u>
  - Services include counseling, medication-assisted treatment, and support groups.

Civilian Resources:

- **Substance Abuse and Mental Health Services Administration (SAMHSA):** Provides a national helpline offering free, confidential information and referrals for individuals facing mental health or substance use disorders.
  - **Call:** 1-800-662-HELP (4357)
  - **Website:** <u>samhsa.gov/find-help/national-helpline</u>
  - The helpline operates 24/7, connecting callers to local treatment facilities, support groups, and community-based organizations.
- **National Institute of Mental Health (NIMH):** Offers resources and information on mental health conditions, including substance use disorders.
  - **Website:** <u>nimh.nih.gov</u>
  - Provides educational materials and guides on finding help and treatment options.

Additional Support:

* **Narcotics Anonymous (NA):** A global, community-based organization offering support for individuals recovering from drug addiction.
    * Website: na.org
    * Provides information on local meetings and recovery resources.
* **Alcoholics Anonymous (AA):** A fellowship of individuals seeking to overcome alcohol addiction through shared experiences and support.
    * Website: aa.org
    * Offers a directory of local meetings and resources for recovery.

Remember, seeking help is a sign of strength. If you or someone you know is in crisis, don't hesitate to reach out to these resources.

ABOUT THE AUTHOR

Matt Arrowood

Well first of all Thank you all for your support!
This is only my first book and I have plenty more planned. I am a five year Army veteran and proud of it! I wrote this book to bring awareness to how many veterans thank and are treated when they first get discharged from any service. I do have a family and a loving wife that encourages my stories and helps me with proof reading. So she's the real hero! My stories are normally horror, military or adventure type. I hope you all are as excited as I am for the future books/stories that are soon to come!

Thank you everyone again for reading and I look forward to sharing more of my stories with you all!!